LIVING WITHOUT FAT:

Practical guide to losing stubborn belly fat for good

Melvin Great

TABLE OF CONTENT

INTRODCTION

Many individuals deal with persistent abdominal fat. It might be tough to find out how to remove your belly fat; it requires time, effort, and patience. There is no quick answer unless you want to submit to pricey surgery like liposuction, which frequently is just a temporary fix without keeping a balanced diet and workout program.

Persistent belly fat must be removed one pound at a time with diet and exercise. There are three basic techniques to remove your belly fat: regular exercise, lower calorie consumption, and abdominal workouts. Mix them and you will have the ingredients for an efficient weight reduction regimen.

To begin to shed your belly fat, you need change your diet. Keep in mind that high-fat, high-calorie meals are a treat, not a daily food category. Take the time to clean up your cabinets and refrigerator and eliminate any of these sorts of goods from your house. If you keep them around, you'll eat them. Contact a specialist to calculate a suitable quantity of calories for weight reduction, and adhere to this regimen. This reduced-calorie diet will help prevent new belly fat from developing up.

Secondly, you need to establish a regular fitness plan. Pick a heart-pumping workout that you love, and include it on a regular basis. You may undertake new things each day if you are easily bored. Make careful, though, to exercise for at least 30 minutes every day. Your body consumes energy from sugar during the first 10-15 minutes when you workout. Only after that does it begin burning the fat around your midsection. The more cardio you perform the more fat you will burn; it's a simple math.

When you have began to shed your belly fat, you'll want to begin a series of abdominal workouts. These workouts will develop your muscles and lead to a slim, toned appearance. You can do them before you drop the fat, but you won't notice any substantial effects until you've shed the appropriate weight. Six-pack abs do you no good if they're hidden by superfluous layers of fat!

CHAPTER ONE

FACTS ABOUT BELLY FAT

A person's general health may be inferred by the size of their stomach. Even individuals who are slim elsewhere may have a potbelly, which makes them seem unhealthy and causes those of us with pot bellies to often feel ill as a result.

When it comes to losing abdominal fat, there are both good and bad news. The good news is that it is possible. You can reduce your belly fat and get in better shape regardless of how large your tummy is or how long you've been overweight.

Unfortunately, there isn't actually a secret or a hack to achieving it. You have undoubtedly seen a variety of methods for reducing abdominal fat for years. Maybe you've tried several approaches—such as various diets and exercise regimens—and either the benefits weren't noticeable right away or you just abandoned the plan.

The bad news is that you probably gave up while you were on the correct track. You may reduce belly fat by combining any healthy food plan with an exercise routine. That may not be interesting or attractive, but you can still attempt it. Finding a strategy that works for you personally is the most difficult step.

Diets that are successful for your coworkers and neighbors may not be successful for you. Everyone is unique. There wouldn't be as many distinct diets that so many different individuals can lose weight with if one strategy worked for everyone. There would be a single strategy for everyone that, if followed, would always be successful.

Alternatively, there are diets that emphasize veggies and are minimal in calories, fat, and carbs. There are a huge variety of specific diets available. This time, avoid starting a diet. Just decide to consume less calories and healthier food than you have been. This will accelerate your fat reduction, and soon you'll have much reduced belly fat.

You can lose belly fat with this alone, just as you may lose fat generally. You will lose fat if you consume less calories than you expend. But, if your form is just different and you have a bigger belly, it could seem like this is where you lose fat the least.

Do activities that specifically target that region to reduce its size and give the impression that you have lost a lot of abdominal fat. You will burn fat more quickly throughout your body if you do thigh-specific strength training workouts. The reason behind this is because increasing the efficiency of your major muscle groups will raise your metabolism.

Also, concentrate on the abdomen region with some crunches and even Pilates and yoga workouts. These workouts will tighten those muscles and reduce the size of your whole abdominal region. Start off slowly to avoid self-harm, and then gradually increase.

You may attain your belly fat reduction objectives much more quickly by doing all of these things, and before you know it, you'll have a lovely tight stomach with all the fat melting away.

CHAPTER TWO

BELLY FAT AND DIABETES (THE CONNECTION)

Do abdominal obesity and diabetes really go hand in hand? Regrettably, there is evidence to suggest that those who have greater body fat in their stomach and other areas are more likely to develop metabolic syndrome. Those with higher belly fat seem to be more susceptible to heart disease, high blood pressure, high cholesterol, and diabetes.

Several body kinds have fruit names. Those with pear-shaped bodies experience these issues far less often than persons with apple-shaped bodies who are overweight above the waist and have round middles. So, if you have a lot of abdominal fat, are you on a one-way train to diabetes that you can't get off of?

Absolutely not. It's unclear if those who have more belly fat are more likely to get diabetes or whether the fat gathers around the center because they were born predisposed to the disease.

In other words, medical professionals and academics are unsure of how metabolic syndrome and belly obesity came to be. Does having fat make you more likely to develop diabetes, or does having fat make you more likely to have it? One thing is clear, however. The risk of developing diabetes is reduced by losing abdominal fat.

In reality, data demonstrate that type II diabetes, often known as adult-onset diabetes, is virtually always avoidable. Juvenile diabetes, a type 1 condition, primarily affects children. This affects young individuals when their pancreas either fails to produce any insulin at all or insufficient amounts.

Being overweight or having belly fat has nothing to do with type 1 diabetes. In contrast, type II diabetes is thought to be mostly brought on by lifestyle choices. The main causes of this condition are thought to primarily be poor eating habits and either no exercise or very little activity.

You may take efforts to attempt to avoid diabetes in yourself even if everyone in your family has the disease. Diabetes is unquestionably a risk for someone who has a lot of abdominal fat. Your risk of developing diabetes may not be immediately impacted by weight loss. You could still be on the path to diabetes even if someone could remove the excess fat from your stomach without you making any lifestyle changes.

Yet, the steps you take to reduce your abdominal fat have such a good impact on your health that they significantly minimize your chance of developing diabetes. Your chance of developing conditions like diabetes, heart disease, high cholesterol, and even knee issues decreases even after dropping only 10 pounds.

Hence, reducing abdominal fat doesn't really change anything. Making good decisions and losing weight are what can prevent you from developing diabetes.

The procedures are easy. Consume complex carbs such as whole grains and oats. Make fruits, vegetables, whole grains, and extremely lean proteins the foundation of your diet. Furthermore, don't forget to exercise often. These smart decisions will help you prevent this chronic and possibly disabling condition because of the link between abdominal obesity and diabetes.

CHAPTER THREE

TWEAK YOUR DIET AND STICK TO IT

Remember that the secret to achieving a flat tummy is to decrease total body fat. The stomach fat is the last to disappear, thus it's the most difficult. Here are a few pointers to assist you get rid of that last bit of stubborn tummy fat.

First and foremost, you must consume more fiber. The main reason individuals, particularly women, are becoming heavier these days is a lack of fiber in their diets. Natural fibers in our diet are getting scarcer as we consume more processed foods and less whole grains and fruits and vegetables. Aim for at least 25 grams of fiber per day for the typical individual. Those who are serious about losing abdominal fat should consume 35 grams of fiber every day.

Second, know that carbs aren't the devil that some diets portray them to be, but that eating too many carbohydrates might enlarge your waistline. Carbohydrates should account for no more than 60% of your calories while on a diet to reduce abdominal fat.

Make them up at least 45 percent of your diet. As you can see, the crucial word here is balance. The majority of your carbohydrates should come from fruits and vegetables, and high-carb, empty-calorie meals like cupcakes should be avoided.

These are some of the finest meals to consider for losing tummy fat:

Fish and other seafood - rich in protein, vital fatty acids, and minerals, these meals aid in the maintenance of a healthy metabolism.

Leafy greens - high in antioxidants and vitamins, leafy green vegetables such as spinach, kale, and arugula may help decrease inflammation caused by extra belly fat.

Berries - high in antioxidants and fiber, berries such as blueberries and raspberries are low in calories but high in taste, so they may help reduce cravings while also delivering nourishment.

Avocados are high in heart-healthy lipids that help keep cholesterol levels in line while also providing important minerals like potassium to ease digestion.

Nuts, which are abundant in protein and healthy fats, may fulfill hunger needs while also increasing fullness.

Beans, which are high in protein and fiber, are also high in complex carbs, which provide energy throughout the day.

Whole grains - It's important to consume whole grain carbohydrates like oats or quinoa to maintain energy levels without generating an insulin rise.

Lastly, drink plenty of water. Many individuals assume that consuming a lot of water would result in bulging abs. Water, on the other hand, flushes salt out of your system, reducing puffiness.

Never go without water for an extended period of time. The color of your urine is one method to tell whether you're dehydrated. If you consume enough water, your urine should be almost white.

Fourth, reduce your salt consumption since it causes puffiness. For the body's natural processes to operate, a person only requires 500 mg of salt each day. You may reduce your salt intake by eating fresh, natural foods.

Finally, prepare a little meal and then close the kitchen. It is critical to consume calories throughout the day while you are actively burning them. Evening eating is often aimless. You plop down in front of the TV with a fresh new bag of chips, and before you know it, half of the bag is gone. Another advantage of eating light at night is that you'll be hungry for a big breakfast in the morning. Good breakfast eaters are more likely to lose weight.

You'll have to follow the advice you've undoubtedly been hearing for years if you want to know how to lose stubborn belly fat. You must follow a healthy dietary plan. Without a healthy eating plan, all of your other efforts will be diminished, and what is the purpose of working hard if you are sabotaging yourself with what you eat?

It's quite simple to do everything properly in terms of fitness yet consume the wrong meals. Regrettably, today's nutritional advice often contradicts itself. This group seems to be doing well despite not eating carbs. Others consume largely carbs and avoid greasy meals. Some don't care about carbohydrates or fats and just check calories.

Several individuals are successful utilizing this strategy in all three of these various groupings. But how can you determine which one is the best fit for you? All you can do is choose one and see whether you can stay with it. If it is not for you, try something else. A healthy diet is often low in carbohydrates and processed foods.

Carbohydrates in diets that do include a lot of them are generally extremely complex carbs. These diets include oatmeal and tiny servings of pasta that have been cooked al dente, which means they are firm and not mushy. Good carb diets emphasize eating carbs that take a long time to digest and maintain your blood sugar steady.

This diet should be suitable for almost everyone. But, if the quantity of carbs is so low that you feel hungry and it doesn't seem right for you, try a higher-carb but low-fat diet. If this kind of diet does not seem to help you lose weight, there are still Weight Watchers and other diets that concentrate on calories.

The most essential thing is to choose one you can rely on. But even the greatest diet in the world will not help you lose weight if you do not stick to it. Eating well may help you reduce weight, which can help you shed fat throughout your body. While it is impossible to concentrate just on belly fat, it is critical to include lots of exercise in your regimen.

CHAPTER FOUR

TIPS TO LOSING BELLY FAT

Developing a balanced food plan is one component of the quickest approach to reduce belly fat. This is a long-term eating strategy, not a fad diet. Yo-yo dieting really exacerbates the stomach fat issue since you lose weight in other places but gain it back in the stomach first. Making a lasting adjustment in your diet is thus critical. You're creating a lifestyle, not just a quick fix.

Your diet should be concerned not only with the overall quantity of calories but also with the types of calories. For every pound you weigh, you should consume at least 1 gram of protein every day. You must also include fat in your diet. A 30:20:50 protein:fat:carbohydrates diet makes a lot of sense for an overweight lady looking for the quickest approach to reduce abdominal fat. Fish oils are the greatest kind of fat for this.

You will lose fat all throughout your body, including your belly. Some diets promise to give you a flat stomach, but it's simply regular weight reduction and perhaps certain dietary choices that reduce abdominal bloating. Consuming meals that aren't gassy or acidic will assist make your stomach seem smaller by reducing gas and bloating.

First and foremost, you should eat a well-balanced low-calorie diet. One idea is to "eat around the perimeter of the store." That example, avoid the isles stocked with processed foods. Consume plenty of fresh fruits and vegetables, as well as lean meat and low-fat dairy products. Increase your intake of natural foods such as whole grains and beans. Avoiding carbonated and sugary drinks, such as soda, may also help you lose weight. Although you will not lose belly fat to make it smaller, it will be less full of food or the gases produced by carbonation and will seem smaller.

Lastly, you must lower your calorie intake. You want to consume 500 less calories than you would normally consume in order to maintain your weight.

GET THAT FAT OFF YOUR CARDIO

Perform cardio workouts like walking, running, or aerobic dancing 4 to 5 times each week to help you burn fat everywhere.

Try yoga or Pilates, which are calm, contemplative movements that strengthen your core abdominal muscles.

The ideal method is to exercise for an hour every other day and strength train for 45 minutes to an hour every other day.

Aerobic workouts include walking, jogging, cycling, and working out on cardio equipment at the gym.

To really grasp how to eliminate lower belly fat, you must first recognize that it is distinct from the rest of your abs. Sit-ups and ab exercises may assist, but they won't cure it. You must exercise cardio in addition to your ab workouts. You may not notice immediate benefits, but persevere.

Hatha Yoga, in addition to sit-ups, may help reduce abdominal fat. Vajrasana exercises require you to bend to the front of your knees, which is an excellent workout. If you are a novice, you should practise this kind of yoga under the supervision of an instructor.

Work with your legs in addition to your tummy muscles. Do movements that demand your legs to be at or above your lower waistline. In order to maintain your equilibrium, your lower abdominal muscles must contract. Kickboxing is an excellent example of an activity that will keep your tummy fully flat.

This kind of leg workout may be obtained by vigorous dancing. It not only helps you reduce weight, but it also tones your legs and helps you shed tummy fat. Belly dance, in particular, will help you lose belly fat. You may either attend a class or watch videos to learn the moves.

Besides from cardio, you should do weight training at least three times each week. Keep in mind that muscular mass burns fat. As you gain muscle, your body burns fat throughout the day, not just when you exercise. Don't overlook this component of decreasing lower abdominal fat.

To get the firm, flat stomach you want, you must first come close to your optimum body weight. Your lower abdominal fat will be one of the last to go. If you are 40-50 pounds overweight, getting in shape should be your first priority, since shedding lower belly fat will only happen until the majority of your other fat is gone. Some forms of activities will help if you are fit and only have a little pouch. But, if you are overweight, it will need some long-term effort.

Crunches are a great way to tighten and work your abs. This will significantly tighten the muscles and make them considerably smaller, so that when you lose weight all around, your stomach will appear substantially different.

Do these workouts in addition to fat-burning routines and a balanced dietary plan. To decrease baby belly fat, try to complete a 45-minute heart-healthy exercise at least three times each week. This may involve running, jogging, cycling, or utilizing any cardio equipment at the gym. Exercising in conjunction with such a diet might help you target certain regions to decrease, like as your tummy.

GET A BALL OF STABILITY

Exercise with a stability ball if you want to reduce abdominal fat. This piece of training equipment might be the deciding factor in your quest for a flat stomach or washboard abs. According to research, persons who worked out using stability boards had twice as many muscle fibers in their bellies as those who just performed crunches. Use a stability ball to do a lose belly fat workout regimen.

These three lose belly fat exercises listed here might help novices get started.

To begin, sit on the ball and lay your hands on it for balance. Alternately, put your hands behind your head for a more harder but more effective strength workout. Begin slowly rolling your hips in a circle to the right, first in tiny circles and then bigger circles as you get more comfortable. Complete 10 to 20 circles, then switch sides and continue the exercise. Although it may seem easy, this exercise will train all of the stomach muscles, making it ideal for losing belly fat.

The Sitting March is the next exercise for losing abdominal fat. Sit on the ball, spine straight and abs tight. Begin a leisurely march by raising the right foot first, then the left. Lift your knees higher and march quicker as you get more comfortable with the activity. If you feel comfortable, you may even apply a bounce to the ball. This exercise should be repeated for 1 to 2 minutes.

The Sitting Balance is the last beginner's exercise I'll go through here. You will sit on the ball, spine straight and abs tight. Lift your right foot off the floor, keeping it in the air for at least 5 seconds if you are a novice, or behind your head if you are more confident. Lower, then repeat on the other side. Repeat 5–10 times more. Maintain your equilibrium by contracting your abs.

Many of these reduce belly fat workout routines for beginners include you sitting on the ball. As you acquire confidence with the stability ball, you will start doing exercises from the floor, your knees, and even resting on top of the ball. The instructions that comes with the stability ball should offer a variety of exercises with graphics to assist you understand what you should be doing. Use an 18-inch ball if you are under 5'1". From 5'1 to 5'8, a 22-inch ball is recommended, while those beyond 5'8 should use a 26-inch ball.

Apart from the procedures mentioned above, the following tactics have been shown to be particularly successful in reducing belly fat:

Do your sit-ups.

Sit-ups and crunches are the simplest and arguably the most efficient strategy to decrease belly fat quickly. You will attain the necessary outcomes in no time. All fat is merely stored energy. Consequently, in order to decrease belly fat, you need to burn more calories than you ingest. In order to achieve the finest results, you need to complete sit-ups, which are the single most effective exercise. They work on practically all body types.

Plank Hold

The plank workout targets Abdominal Muscles, Shoulders, Back Muscles, Chest Muscles, Glutes. It is a wonderful workout for slimming down tummy fat.

Steps

Start by getting into a push up posture with your hands and feet on the floor, just below your shoulders and hips respectively; making sure to maintain your spine neutral throughout the whole action!

After you're in this posture, proceed to drag your belly button in towards your spine while keeping a straight line from your head all the way down to your heels—very critical for optimal results!

Maintain this stance for 30 seconds (or longer, depending on individual fitness level) while keeping perfect form throughout. Don't forget to breathe deeply while holding the pose—it could assist distract you from any pain or stiffness you may encounter during plank!

After time's up, gently come back down into starting position and relax momentarily before trying another set or going on to other exercises. Remember, form is vital here so be sure not to hurry through this one - slow and controlled movements are important as they will assist guarantee both safety as well as efficacy of workout!

Crunches

This will concentrate on your Lower Abs, Middle Abs, Rhomboids, Glutes, and Obliques.

Steps

Lay flat on your back, with your legs bent at the knees and feet resting on the ground. Ensure that there is no unnecessary strain on your lower back when executing this exercise.

Put both hands behind your head, with your elbows pointed outwards. Maintain a tiny space between your chin and chest throughout the exercise—this will assist you remain in perfect form when you crunch!

Now, utilizing solely your abdominal muscles, engage and push yourself up towards the sky until you feel a nice contraction in your abdominal region—your shoulder blades should be off the ground at this point while still maintaining your neck aligned with your spine throughout the exercise.

Pause briefly before gently lowering yourself back down toward starting position in a controlled manner—this aspect of the action functions as eccentric loading for muscle growth so be sure not to hurry through it!

Continue for the appropriate number of repetitions; rest momentarily between sets if required before going on to other exercises or onto the next round of crunches!

Squats

This workout targets your Quads, Glutes, Hamstrings, Core Muscles, and Calves.

Steps

Begin by standing with your feet shoulder-width apart, toes looking straight forward, and back straight throughout the whole exercise. Be careful to maintain your chest up and head in a neutral position—this will help you remain in perfect form.

Gently continue to engage the core muscles while engaging and pulling the hips back (like sitting down in an imagined chair) until both thighs reach parallel with the ground. Be cautious not to sink too low into the squat; maintain the bulk of your weight on heels throughout movement!

At this point, stop briefly before pushing through your heels to bring yourself up towards starting position in one continuous motion—make sure to maintain your core engaged throughout this section of the action!

Continue for the appropriate number of repetitions; rest momentarily between sets if required before proceeding onto other exercises or another round of squats.

Knee High

These workouts need quick twitch muscle fibers which implies higher energy expenditure over intervals compared to static postures like planking, making them the best alternative when seeking to blast away extra belly fat remaining around the waistline region.

Target regions include Quads, Glutes, Hamstrings, Core Muscles, Calves, Cardiovascular System

Steps

Start by standing with your feet shoulder-width apart and your core engaged throughout the action.

With the body erect and your eyes ahead, swiftly raise the left leg up towards the chest while simultaneously extending the right arm forward as far as possible while maintaining the elbow straight (like a racing stride).

From here, immediately swap arms and legs before bringing the right knee up towards the chest while pushing off the left leg forcefully, keeping both feet off the ground at all times.

Perform this action for the appropriate amount of repetitions or seconds, keeping a consistent, steady tempo throughout each rep!

If necessary, take a short break between sets before moving on to other exercises or another round of high knees.

Remove the fried items.

Certain meals must be avoided in order to have a flat stomach. Fried meals will increase belly fat quicker than any other calorie consumption. Fried meals are largely made up of empty calories with little nutritional value. They merely supply calories, which contribute to belly fat.

Avoid snacking in between meals.

Snacking is one of the finest (or worst) ways to pack on the pounds. Late-night munching is the worst kind of snacking. As you ingest calories throughout the day, you have the opportunity to burn them off. When you eat at night, you retire to bed, and the food just sits in your stomach.

Moreover, when you eat at night, you are more likely to indulge in mindless snacking. You'll start with a complete bag of chips and within an hour of watching television, half of them will be gone. When you snack, you are not paying attention to what you are eating, which forces you to remark, "I want to lose my belly fat."

That should be burned away.

As previously said, belly fat is useless energy. It builds up in the form of fat in the stomach. If you want to lose belly fat, you must burn more calories than you consume. Aerobic exercise of any type is beneficial for losing abdominal fat. Walking, jogging, cycling, or working out on a cardio machine at the gym are all examples. Even simple things like taking the stairs at work instead of the elevator or parking in the furthest spot while heading to the mall may assist.

HOW TO LOSE BELLY FAT

Many individuals make the process of losing excess belly fat needlessly complex. The good news is that you don't have to watch countless fitness videos, read hundreds of books, or do a dozen different types of exercises to lose belly fat. Just follow these few instructions.

As previously said, it is critical to understand that reducing belly fat entails burning fat throughout your whole body.

Spot exercising or spot reduction refers to attempting to target certain portions of your body. It is not functional. To lose belly fat, you must first follow an effective overall fat-burning regimen.

This strategy will assist you in doing so.

Determine Your Maximum Heart Rate

Your maximal heart rate is the fastest your heart can beat if you push yourself really hard during a workout. It is not good to continuously push yourself to your utmost pace.

Knowing your maximal heart rate, on the other hand, can help you establish a goal for how hard you want to work out.

Workout at 70% of your target heart rate on a regular basis.

You can find out your heart rate on almost every workout equipment at the gym. If you don't want to utilize gym equipment, you may simply get a heart rate monitor.

By monitoring your activity in terms of heart rate rather than distance ran or time spent exercising, you may compare yourself to other persons your age and weight.

Should you feel happy or awful for running "just" 20 minutes? It's difficult to say since time is a lousy measure. Instead, knowing your goal heart rate allows you to push yourself while also seeing how well you're doing overall.

Decrease your intake of fat and sodium.

Even if you exercise consistently, losing belly fat will be tough if you do not lower your calorie and salt consumption.

Begin by reducing your calorie intake. Don't attempt to accomplish everything at once; instead, progressively reduce your intake of high-calorie items.

Reduce the quantity of salt you consume in your diet. Sodium is important in controlling how much water your body stores in fat cells and the circulation. Increased salt consumption results in fatter cells and increased blood pressure.

These three procedures, when followed consistently, are all that is required to burn abdominal fat. You don't need complicated methods or fad diets; all you need is some self-discipline to stay with the system.

This approach will assist you in determining how hard you need to work out and maintain your heart rate at that level in order to drop enough weight to burn abdominal fat. It will also assist you in maintaining your weight loss via regular dieting.

Protein might be the most significant macronutrient for losing weight. It has been shown to lower cravings by 60%, increase metabolism by 80-100 calories per day, and assist you in eating up to 441 less calories each day.

If you want to lose weight, adding protein to your diet may be one of the most beneficial improvements you can make. Protein may not only help you lose weight, but it can also assist you prevent regaining weight. Increase your protein intake by eating more high-protein foods such whole eggs, seafood, legumes, nuts, meat, and dairy products.

CHAPTER FIVE

BENEFITS OF LOSING THAT BELLY FAT

Improved sleep

Snoozing certainly helped you lose more weight in the first place, but as a consequence of your weight reduction you'll actually get higher quality sleep today. Studies reveals that decreasing 5% of your bodyweight will help you sleep better and longer throughout the night. What's more, purging your body of extra fat may also help cure sleep apnea and snoring.

Improved hormonal balance

When you think of hormones, your teenage years may rush to mind, but they play a role in more than simply your developing sex desire throughout puberty. The thyroid gland manufactures and releases two extremely essential hormones which govern your metabolism and may also impact muscular strength among other things. As you clear your body of extra fat your hormones stabilize and as a consequence it's simpler for you to sustain or even further your weight reduction,

Enhanced sex drive

Too tired? Not anymore. Soon you don't have to think twice about getting in the mood, and you may find yourself intentionally holding yourself back from going for round three. Weight reduction is connected to improved testosterone levels and an increased libido, and reducing only 10 pounds is enough to trigger sex hormones. What's more, fitting in your exercise every morning also boosts blood flow to the pelvic region, further enhancing your desire.

Improved mood

Committing to the gym may have pushed your body to the point it is today, but it also boosted your mental health. Working exercise generates feel-good molecules called endorphins. Endorphins are responsible for the high you get post-workout. They interact with the receptors in your brain, lowering your experience of pain, and produce a good sensation in the body comparable to that of morphine.

Decreased joint pain

Your joints already take a battering from regular wear and tear—extra weight hanging around on your belly simply makes things worse. Simply simply, the less you weigh the less your skeletal system and joints have to support, which translates into less joint discomfort.

Clearer, brighter skin

You may have begun your healthy regimen with the sole purpose of slimming down, but an extra advantage of your weight-loss journey comes in the shape of glowing skin. You may owe your improved complexion to the boost in nutrients from all the fruits and vegetables you're likely consuming and also to all that sweat physically forcing the trash out of your pores, supporting better detoxification, says Smith. Just be sure to cleanse your face periodically after your exercise activity to prevent unsightly breakouts and congested pores.

Stress alleviation

If you ticked off losing weight from your to-do list, you've already got one less item to fret about. Seriously however, the things you do to lose weight—eating a balanced diet, exercising frequently, and getting plenty of sleep—are also some of the finest strategies to decrease tension and anxiety.

CONCLUSION

From what you have learnt it this book, one thin is obvious. There's hope for you. No matter how long you've been overweight, you can still shed that fat and acquire that mouth watering form you so want.

On one hand, it falls totally on you. In other words, you are the architect of your own weight destiny. The decisions you make will go a long way to decide where your weight reduction journey finish up. Weight reduction, particularly belly fat demands discipline and determination.

This book has been meticulously designed to assist you reach your objectives but it will be like every other weight loss book you've read in the past if you don't make the choice to work and push yourself.

I urge you to take the action and watch how you change into the person you've always wanted to be.

www.ingramcontent.com/pod-product-compliance
Lightning Source LLC
Chambersburg PA
CBHW061606250726

48657CB00017B/2111